Embrace the Glucose Revolution

Ignite Your Health, Happiness, and Vitality

by

Theresa D. Shockey

Copyright © 2023 by Theresa D. Shockey

The Glucose Revolution: Transform Your Health and Reclaim Your Vitality is a work of passion, dedication, and transformation. It is a culmination of extensive research, personal experiences, and heartfelt stories aimed at empowering readers to take control of their health and well-being. The information and strategies provided within this book are intended for educational purposes and should not replace professional medical advice. The author and publisher disclaim any liability or responsibility for any adverse effects resulting directly or indirectly from the use or application of the information contained in this book.

Table of Contents

Dedication

To all those who have faced the challenges of imbalanced blood sugar and yearned for a healthier, more vibrant life. This book is dedicated to your unwavering spirit, resilience, and commitment to reclaiming your vitality. May the pages within ignite a spark of inspiration and guide you towards a path of profound transformation and well-being.

Introduction

Prepare yourself for a life-changing adventure where the power of stable blood sugar unlocks a world of virtually endless possibilities. The journey described in "Embrace the Glucose Revolution" is more than just a book; it will hold your attention from start to finish.

Imagine living a life free from cravings, where chronic fatigue is a thing of the past, and where vibrant health and limitless energy are your new normal. The secret to that extraordinary life—a life brimming with vigor, joy, and radiant well-being—lies in this book.

You will be enthralled by tales of resiliency, transformation, and personal growth as you read the moving accounts of people who overcame the difficulties of blood sugar imbalance. As you watch them struggle, have doubts, and ultimately succeed, prepare yourself for a roller coaster of emotions.

You'll learn the techniques for controlling blood sugar levels, getting rid of cravings, and taking back control of your health and happiness with each page you turn. It's an engaging investigation into the relationship between the mind and body, filled with cutting-edge scientific knowledge and doable tactics that will enable you to embrace long-lasting change.

Immerse yourself in this extraordinary journey and prepare to be inspired, moved, and motivated.

More than just a book, "Embrace the Glucose Revolution" opens the door to a life of liberty, joy, and limitless potential. Get ready to embrace the adventure of a lifetime and unleash your inner Glucose Goddess!

Chapter 1
The Glucose Roller Coaster

Think of a roller coaster with its thrilling peaks and jaw-dropping valleys. Now use that comparison to describe how our bodies levels of glucose change throughout the day. The constant rise and fall of blood sugar, which causes energy swings that impact our daily lives, is called the "glucose roller coaster."

Our bodies convert foods high in carbohydrates into glucose, which is absorbed into our bloodstream when we eat them. This results in a sharp rise in blood sugar levels, which gives you an energy boost and a fleeting feeling of well-being. However, this increase is transient, and as our bodies produce insulin to control blood sugar, our energy levels decline.

Cravings and the Cost of Emotion

Our emotions and cravings are some of the most noticeable effects of the glucose roller coaster. After an initial spike in blood sugar, we frequently experience strong cravings for foods high in sugar or carbohydrates. These cravings develop as our bodies look for a temporary fix to raise glucose levels and feel temporarily satisfied.

Cravings can have a high emotional cost. As the satisfaction gained from giving in to cravings is quickly replaced by feelings of regret and dissatisfaction, we may find ourselves caught in a cycle of indulgence and guilt. This emotional roller coaster can harm our health, resulting in low self-esteem and a tense relationship with food.

Chronic Tiredness

Chronic fatigue is another effect of the glucose roller coaster. Our energy levels fluctuate throughout the day as blood sugar levels do. We experience a noticeable loss of energy when our blood glucose levels fall, leaving us exhausted, lazy, and mentally clouded.

It is difficult to maintain consistent vitality due to the constant cycle of energy peaks and crashes, which makes it difficult to remain focused and productive all day. Chronic fatigue impacts many areas of our lives, including our ability to perform well at work and participate in fulfilling activities and relationships.

Taking Charge

It's time to take charge now that we know how the glucose roller coaster affects our health and happiness. We can control blood sugar levels and lessen the effects of these fluctuations by choosing our diet and lifestyle wisely.

Adopting a well-balanced, nutritious diet that prioritizes whole foods, complex carbohydrates, lean proteins, and healthy fats is one strategy for controlling the glucose roller coaster. Regular physical activity, such as strength training and aerobic exercise, can improve insulin sensitivity and help control blood sugar levels.

Awareness of the emotional triggers that lead to cravings and emotional eating is also crucial. The emotional toll of the glucose roller coaster can be lessened by practicing mindful eating, learning stress management techniques, and getting support from medical professionals or support groups.

Chapter 2

Igniting Vitality: Unleashing Your Energy

Understanding Blood Sugar Balance

Blood sugar, or glucose, is the primary source of energy for our bodies. It is obtained through the breakdown of carbohydrates consumed in our diet. However, maintaining optimal blood sugar levels is vital for sustained energy throughout the day. When our blood sugar levels fluctuate too much, it can lead to energy crashes, mood swings, and an overall sense of fatigue.

The Role of Insulin

Insulin, a hormone produced by the pancreas, plays a critical role in regulating blood sugar levels. When we consume carbohydrates, our body releases insulin to facilitate the absorption of glucose into our cells. This process helps maintain stable blood sugar levels, preventing spikes and crashes in energy.

Impact of Imbalanced Blood Sugar

When our blood sugar levels become imbalanced, either due to excessive carbohydrate intake or impaired insulin function, it can have several negative consequences on our energy levels. Elevated blood sugar levels can result in a rapid energy surge followed by a crash, leaving us feeling drained and lethargic. On the other hand, consistently low blood sugar levels can lead to chronic fatigue and reduced stamina.

Nutritional Strategies for Blood Sugar Balance

Maintaining blood sugar balance requires a well-rounded approach that involves making informed dietary choices. Some key strategies include:

a. Consuming Complex Carbohydrates: opt for whole grains, legumes, and vegetables that release glucose slowly into the bloodstream, providing a steady supply of energy.

b. Balancing Macronutrients: Include a combination of carbohydrates, proteins, and healthy fats in your meals to slow down the digestion and absorption of glucose, preventing blood sugar spikes.

c. Portion Control: Moderation is essential when it comes to carbohydrate intake. Be mindful of portion sizes and aim for balanced meals to avoid overwhelming your body with excess glucose.

d. Fiber-Rich Foods: Incorporate fiber-rich foods such as fruits, vegetables, and whole grains into your diet. Fiber helps regulate blood sugar levels by slowing down the absorption of glucose and promoting a feeling of fullness.

e. Regular Meal Timing: Establish a consistent meal schedule to keep blood sugar levels stable throughout the day. Avoid skipping meals, as this can disrupt your energy balance.

Emotional Testimonials of Reclaimed Vitality

Alongside the scientific understanding of blood sugar balance, numerous individuals have experienced transformative improvements in their energy levels and overall vitality by implementing these strategies. Here are a few emotional testimonials from individuals who have successfully reclaimed their energy:

Testimonial 1: John, a 40-year-old executive, shares how making conscious changes to his diet and prioritizing blood sugar balance has led to a significant increase in his energy levels and improved focus at work.

Testimonial 2: Sarah, a busy mother of two, describes how addressing her blood sugar imbalances has helped her maintain steady energy throughout the day, enabling her to better engage with her children and pursue her own interests.

Testimonial 3: Michael, a fitness enthusiast, explains how adopting a diet focused on blood sugar balance has not only enhanced his physical performance but also positively impacted his mental clarity and overall well-being.

Chapter 3

Conquering Cravings: Regaining Control

Examining the Psychological and Emotional Factors Driving Cravings

Cravings can be powerful and challenging to resist, often leading us to indulge in specific foods or substances. While physiological factors like hunger and nutrient deficiencies can trigger cravings, it is essential to understand the psychological and emotional factors that contribute to their intensity.

Psychological Factors

a. Habitual Associations: Cravings frequently arise from the power of associations. Our brains establish connections between certain activities, environments, or emotions and the consumption of particular foods or substances. For instance, if we consistently eat ice cream while watching movies, the act of watching a movie alone can trigger cravings for ice cream. Breaking these associations is key to managing cravings effectively.

b. Conditioning and Rewards: Our brains are wired to seek pleasure and reward. When we consume foods or substances that provide pleasurable sensations, our brains form strong associations between the experience and positive emotions. Over time, these associations contribute to cravings as our brains seek the reward and pleasure associated with the desired item.

c. Emotional Eating: Emotions such as stress, boredom, loneliness, or sadness can trigger cravings as a coping mechanism. Comfort foods, often high in sugar or unhealthy fats, may provide temporary relief or distraction from emotional discomfort. The act of consuming these foods can create a cycle of emotional eating and cravings, further impacting our well-being.

Emotional Factors

a. Emotional Triggers: Emotional factors, such as stress, anxiety, or even positive emotions like excitement or celebration, can stimulate cravings. Stress, in particular, leads to cravings for high-fat, high-sugar foods due to the release of stress hormones affecting appetite regulation. Emotional triggers can vary from person to person, highlighting the importance of recognizing and addressing individual emotional connections to cravings.

b. Mood Enhancement: Certain foods or substances can temporarily alter our mood and provide a sense of comfort or pleasure.

Cravings driven by emotional factors often stem from the desire to experience these mood-altering effects and seek emotional relief or gratification. Understanding these underlying emotional drivers is crucial in effectively managing and overcoming cravings.

c. Coping Mechanisms: Cravings can serve as coping mechanisms to deal with emotional distress. The act of consuming desired foods or substances may provide a sense of control, distraction, or a soothing effect, temporarily alleviating emotional discomfort. Identifying healthier coping mechanisms and developing emotional resilience can help break the cycle of relying on cravings as a means of emotional regulation.

Strategies to Overcome Cravings and Build a Healthier Relationship with Food

Mindful Eating

Mindful eating is a powerful strategy that involves paying full attention to the eating experience. By slowing down and savoring each bite, individuals can develop a deeper awareness of their body's signals of hunger and fullness. Practicing mindful eating allows for a greater understanding of the underlying reasons behind cravings and helps individuals make conscious choices that align with their nutritional needs.

How to achieve this:

- Practice eating slowly and savoring each bite.
- Pay attention to hunger and fullness cues.
- Minimize distractions while eating, such as TV or screens.
- Engage all the senses in the eating experience.

Food Exploration

Engaging in food exploration is a unique strategy that encourages individuals to expand their culinary horizons and discover new flavors and ingredients. Exploring different cuisines, trying exotic fruits or vegetables, or experimenting with unfamiliar recipes can bring excitement and novelty to meals. By diversifying the range of foods consumed, individuals can reduce the monotony that often leads to cravings and foster a more fulfilling and nourishing relationship with food.

How to achieve this:

- Try new recipes and experiment with different ingredients.
- Explore various cuisines and cultural dishes.
- Visit local markets or specialty stores for unique food options.
- Incorporate seasonal and locally sourced produce.

Intuitive Eating

Intuitive eating is an approach that emphasizes listening to the body's cues and honoring its true needs. It involves recognizing and respecting hunger and fullness signals, as well as identifying emotional triggers that may lead to cravings. By reconnecting with the body's innate wisdom and allowing it to guide food choices, individuals can develop a more balanced and intuitive relationship with food, reducing the occurrence of intense cravings.

How to achieve this:

- Listen to your body's hunger and fullness signals.
- Identify emotional triggers that may lead to cravings.
- Practice self-compassion and non-judgment towards food choices.
- Trust your body's wisdom and make choices based on its needs.

Stress Management

Stress is a common trigger for cravings, particularly for comfort foods high in sugar or unhealthy fats. Implementing effective stress management techniques can help individuals address the root causes of cravings. Engaging in activities such as exercise, meditation, or engaging hobbies can provide healthy outlets for stress reduction.

Additionally, practicing self-care, getting sufficient sleep, and seeking support from loved ones can contribute to overall well-being and minimize the reliance on food to cope with stress.

How to achieve this:

- Engage in regular exercise to reduce stress levels.
- Incorporate relaxation techniques such as meditation or deep breathing.
- Prioritize self-care activities that promote relaxation and well-being.
- Seek support from friends, family, or a therapist when needed.

Cognitive Restructuring

Cognitive restructuring involves challenging and reframing the thoughts and beliefs associated with cravings. Instead of viewing cravings as overwhelming and uncontrollable, individuals can adopt a more empowered perspective. By recognizing that cravings are temporary sensations and that they have the ability to make conscious choices, individuals can reframe their mindset and develop a sense of control over their cravings. This approach promotes self-efficacy and a positive outlook in managing and overcoming cravings.

How to achieve this:

- Identify and challenge negative thoughts and beliefs about cravings.
- Reframe cravings as temporary sensations that can be managed.
- Focus on empowering thoughts and beliefs about making conscious choices.
- Use positive affirmations to reinforce a positive mindset.

Mind-Body Techniques

Incorporating mind-body techniques such as yoga, tai chi, or deep breathing exercises can help individuals cultivate a greater sense of mindfulness and emotional balance. These practices promote self-awareness, reduce stress, and increase the ability to respond to cravings in a calm and centered manner. By integrating mind-body techniques into daily routines, individuals can develop resilience in the face of cravings and make more intentional choices aligned with their well-being.

How to achieve this:

- Incorporate regular yoga or tai chi practice for mindfulness and stress reduction.
- Practice deep breathing exercises throughout the day.
- Engage in activities that promote relaxation and mind-body connection.
- Find techniques that resonate with you and integrate them into your routine.

Supportive Environment

Creating a supportive environment is essential for successfully overcoming cravings and building a healthier relationship with food. Surrounding oneself with individuals who share similar goals and values can provide encouragement and accountability. Additionally, removing triggers from the environment, such as keeping unhealthy snacks out of sight or replacing them with nourishing options, can contribute to making healthier choices and reducing the occurrence of cravings.

How to achieve this:

- Surround yourself with supportive individuals who share similar goals.
- Communicate your needs and goals to friends and family.
- Create a home environment that promotes healthy eating choices.
- Seek out support groups or communities that can provide accountability and encouragement.

Chapter 4
Radiant Wellness: Nurturing Your Skin

The condition of our skin is influenced by various factors, including genetics, lifestyle choices, and environmental factors. However, emerging research suggests that blood sugar levels can also play a significant role in skin health.

Exploring the Link between Blood Sugar Levels and Skin Health

Our skin is a complex organ that requires a delicate balance of nutrients and optimal cellular function to maintain its health and vitality. Surprisingly, blood sugar levels play a significant role in skin health. When blood sugar levels are elevated, it triggers a cascade of biochemical reactions that can have a detrimental impact on our skin.

High blood sugar levels lead to a process called glycation, where excess glucose molecules bind to proteins, including collagen and elastin, which are essential for maintaining the structure and elasticity of our skin. This process results in the formation of advanced glycation end products (AGEs), which can contribute to skin aging, wrinkles, and a loss of firmness.

Moreover, elevated blood sugar levels can also trigger inflammation in the body, including the skin. Inflammation disrupts the natural balance of our skin and can contribute to various skin conditions such as acne, eczema, and psoriasis. Furthermore, high blood sugar levels can impair the skin's ability to heal and regenerate, prolonging the recovery time from wounds and skin damage.

Impact of High Blood Sugar on Skin Health

a. Accelerated Aging: High blood sugar levels can contribute to the formation of advanced glycation end products (AGEs) in the body. AGEs can damage collagen and elastin, proteins responsible for skin elasticity and firmness. This process can lead to premature aging, including the development of wrinkles, sagging skin, and loss of radiance.

b. Inflammation and Skin Conditions: Elevated blood sugar levels can trigger chronic inflammation in the body, which may manifest as various skin conditions. Conditions such as acne, eczema, and psoriasis have been linked to inflammation and oxidative stress caused by high blood sugar levels.

c. Impaired Wound Healing: High blood sugar levels can hinder the skin's ability to heal wounds effectively. Elevated glucose levels can impair blood circulation, decrease immune function, and affect the production of growth factors necessary for proper wound healing. This can lead to delayed wound healing and an increased risk of infection.

Strategies for Maintaining Healthy Blood Sugar Levels and Skin Health

a. Balanced Diet: Adopting a balanced diet with a focus on whole foods, low glycemic index carbohydrates, lean proteins, and healthy fats can help regulate blood sugar levels. Include plenty of fruits, vegetables, whole grains, and lean proteins while limiting processed foods, sugary snacks, and refined carbohydrates.

b. Regular Physical Activity: Engaging in regular exercise can improve insulin sensitivity and help regulate blood sugar levels. Aim for a combination of cardiovascular exercise and strength training to reap the maximum benefits for both blood sugar control and overall skin health.

c. Stress Management: Chronic stress can contribute to elevated blood sugar levels. Implement stress management techniques such as meditation, yoga, deep breathing exercises, or engaging in hobbies to reduce stress and support healthy blood sugar regulation.

d. Adequate Sleep: Prioritize getting enough quality sleep as it plays a role in blood sugar regulation. Poor sleep patterns and insufficient sleep have been associated with increased blood sugar levels and impaired insulin sensitivity.

e. Skincare Routine: Establishing a regular skincare routine that includes gentle cleansing, moisturizing, and sun protection can help maintain overall skin health. Incorporate products with antioxidants, such as vitamins C and E, to counteract oxidative stress caused by high blood sugar levels.

Achieving Radiant Skin

The key to nurturing radiant skin lies in maintaining stable blood sugar levels through balanced nutrition. By adopting a diet that promotes blood sugar balance, we can support the health and vitality of our skin.

Choosing whole foods that are rich in antioxidants, vitamins, minerals, and healthy fats is essential for promoting skin health. Antioxidants help protect our skin from oxidative stress and free radicals, which can accelerate aging. These can be found in colorful fruits and vegetables, such as berries, leafy greens, and citrus fruits.

Additionally, including foods that have a low glycemic index, such as whole grains, legumes, and lean proteins, can help regulate blood sugar levels. These foods are digested more slowly, providing a gradual release of glucose into the bloodstream and preventing rapid spikes in blood sugar.

Hydration is also crucial for maintaining healthy skin. Drinking an adequate amount of water helps keep our skin hydrated and supports its natural processes, such as detoxification and regeneration.

Heartwarming Stories of Individuals Who Achieved Radiant Skin Through Balanced Nutrition

These inspiring stories highlight the powerful connection between a well-rounded diet and radiant skin, demonstrating how healthy eating habits can contribute to a glowing complexion and boost overall self-confidence.

Sarah's Journey to Clear Skin

Sarah had struggled with acne for years and had tried numerous skincare products with limited success. Frustrated, she decided to take a holistic approach and revamped her diet. She eliminated processed foods, refined sugars, and dairy products, and instead focused on consuming nutrient-dense foods. Sarah incorporated plenty of fruits, vegetables, whole grains, lean proteins, and healthy fats into her meals. Over time, she noticed a remarkable improvement in her skin. Her acne gradually cleared up, and her complexion became radiant and healthy. Sarah's story is a testament to the transformative power of balanced nutrition on skin health.

Mark's Radiant Transformation

Mark had dealt with dull and lackluster skin for years. He had tried various skincare routines and treatments but saw minimal improvement. Seeking a more sustainable solution, Mark decided to make dietary changes. He started incorporating antioxidant-rich foods into his meals, such as berries, leafy greens, and nuts. Additionally, he increased his intake of omega-3 fatty acids by consuming fatty fish, chia seeds, and flaxseeds. Over time, Mark's skin began to glow with vitality. The combination of antioxidants and healthy fats in his diet nourished his skin from within, resulting in a radiant transformation.

Emma's Journey to a Youthful Glow

Emma had noticed signs of aging on her skin, including fine lines and loss of elasticity. Determined to address these concerns naturally, she focused on consuming foods with anti-aging properties. Emma incorporated collagen-boosting foods, such as bone broth, citrus fruits, and leafy greens, into her diet. She also included foods rich in antioxidants, such as tomatoes, avocados, and green tea. Over time, Emma's skin regained its youthful glow, and the appearance of fine lines diminished significantly. Her dedication to a balanced diet rich in skin-loving nutrients had remarkable anti-aging effects.

Jason's Journey to Skin Healing

Jason had struggled with eczema, a chronic inflammatory skin condition, for most of his life. Tired of relying solely on topical treatments, he decided to explore the impact of his diet on his skin. Jason eliminated potential trigger foods, such as gluten, dairy, and processed sugars, from his meals. Instead, he focused on consuming anti-inflammatory foods like fatty fish, turmeric, and leafy greens. To his amazement, Jason's eczema flare-ups reduced in frequency and intensity. His skin became calmer, less itchy, and more hydrated. Jason's journey demonstrates how targeted dietary changes can significantly impact skin conditions like eczema.

Chapter 5

Embracing the Fountain of Youth: Aging Gracefully

Aging is an inevitable part of life, but by understanding the impact of blood sugar on our bodies and minds, we can take proactive steps to embrace the fountain of youth. Through the unveiling of scientific insights and inspiring anecdotes of individuals who have defied age through glucose management, we embark on a journey toward vibrant and graceful aging.

The Impact of Blood Sugar on Aging

High blood sugar levels can accelerate the aging process, both internally and externally. When blood sugar remains elevated for prolonged periods, it triggers a series of chemical reactions that can have detrimental effects on our cells, tissues, and organs.

One of the key processes influenced by blood sugar is glycation. Elevated blood sugar levels can lead to the formation of advanced glycation end products (AGEs). These AGEs can accumulate in our cells and tissues, causing damage to proteins, lipids, and DNA. This process contributes to the development of age-related conditions such as cardiovascular diseases, neurodegenerative disorders, and skin aging.

Moreover, high blood sugar levels can also lead to chronic inflammation, a state of persistent immune response. Chronic inflammation accelerates the aging process and increases the risk of developing various age-related diseases, including arthritis, diabetes, and certain types of cancer.

Inspiring Anecdotes of Individuals Who Defied Age through Glucose Management

Interwoven within the scientific understanding of blood sugar and aging are inspiring anecdotes of individuals who have embraced the path of graceful aging through effective glucose management. These personal stories highlight the transformative power of maintaining stable blood sugar levels and making conscious choices to support overall health.

Maria's Remarkable Energy at 70

Maria, a vibrant 70-year-old, credits her high energy levels and youthful appearance to her diligent glucose management. She adopted a low glycemic index diet, focusing on whole foods, complex carbohydrates, lean proteins, and healthy fats. By avoiding processed sugars and refined carbohydrates, Maria maintained stable blood sugar levels throughout the day. As a result, she experienced sustained energy levels, improved mental clarity, and better physical stamina. Maria's inspiring journey demonstrates how effective glucose management can defy age and enable individuals to embrace an active and fulfilling lifestyle.

Robert's Cognitive Vitality at 80

At the age of 80, Robert remains mentally sharp and engaged, thanks to his dedication to glucose management. He follows a Mediterranean-style diet, which emphasizes fresh fruits, vegetables, whole grains, fish, and olive oil. By prioritizing nutrient-dense foods and minimizing sugary treats, Robert maintains stable blood sugar levels, reducing the risk of cognitive decline. His commitment to glucose management has allowed him to preserve his cognitive function, memory, and overall mental well-being, defying age-related cognitive challenges.

Lisa's Vibrant Appearance at 60

Lisa, a 60-year-old with radiant skin and a youthful appearance, attributes her age-defying looks to her diligent glucose management. She adopted a balanced diet that includes plenty of antioxidants, such as berries, leafy greens, and colorful vegetables. Lisa also practices regular physical activity to support insulin sensitivity and maintain healthy blood sugar levels. Her commitment to glucose management has contributed to healthy skin, reduced inflammation, and a youthful glow. Lisa's story serves as an inspiration for individuals looking to defy age and maintain a vibrant appearance through effective glucose control.

James' Robust Health at 90

At the age of 90, James continues to enjoy robust health and an active lifestyle, all thanks to his meticulous glucose management. He follows a well-balanced diet that includes controlled portions, fiber-rich foods, and regular meals throughout the day. By carefully managing his carbohydrate intake, James maintains stable blood sugar levels, reducing the risk of age-related health conditions such as diabetes and cardiovascular disease. His commitment to glucose management has allowed him to enjoy a high quality of life, defying the limitations often associated with advanced age.

Through their journeys, we witness individuals who have adopted healthy dietary practices, engaged in regular physical activity, and implemented stress management techniques. These efforts have resulted in remarkable improvements in their physical appearance, cognitive function, energy levels, and overall quality of life. Their stories serve as beacons of hope and motivation, demonstrating that aging gracefully is within reach for anyone willing to take charge of their blood sugar levels.

Strategies for Graceful Aging

To embrace the fountain of youth and promote graceful aging, it is essential to adopt strategies that prioritize blood sugar management and overall well-being.

Balanced Nutrition: A diet rich in whole foods, including fiber-rich carbohydrates, lean proteins, and healthy fats, can support blood sugar stability. Incorporating antioxidant-rich fruits and vegetables, along with foods high in omega-3 fatty acids, can help combat inflammation and protect against age-related damage.

Physical Activity: Regular exercise, including aerobic activities, strength training, and flexibility exercises, can promote healthy blood sugar levels, improve cardiovascular health, enhance muscle strength, and support overall vitality. Finding enjoyable activities that suit individual preferences and abilities is key to maintaining consistency.

Stress Management: Chronic stress can elevate blood sugar levels and accelerate the aging process. Implementing stress management techniques such as mindfulness meditation, deep breathing exercises, and engaging in hobbies or activities that bring joy and relaxation can support healthy aging.

Sleep Optimization: Quality sleep is crucial for cellular repair, hormone regulation, and overall rejuvenation.

Prioritizing a consistent sleep schedule, creating a sleep-friendly environment, and practicing relaxation techniques can contribute to restorative rest and graceful aging.

Chapter 6

Restful Rejuvenation: The Power of Sleep

Sleep is a vital component of our overall well-being, influencing our physical, mental, and emotional health. By delving into the scientific mechanisms at play and uncovering personal narratives of transformed sleep patterns, we unlock the power of restful rejuvenation for a more energized and vibrant life.

Deep-diving into the Connection between Blood Sugar Stability and Quality Sleep

Sleep and blood sugar levels are intricately interconnected, with each influencing the other in a bidirectional manner. Disruptions in blood sugar stability can lead to poor sleep, while inadequate or poor-quality sleep can affect blood sugar regulation.

When blood sugar levels are imbalanced, particularly elevated, it can interfere with our ability to achieve restorative sleep. High blood sugar triggers an increase in insulin production, which can cause fluctuations in blood sugar levels throughout the night.

These fluctuations can disrupt the normal sleep cycle, leading to frequent awakenings, difficulty falling asleep, or restless sleep.

Conversely, insufficient or poor-quality sleep can impair our body's ability to regulate blood sugar effectively. Sleep deprivation can lead to insulin resistance, a condition where our cells become less responsive to insulin, resulting in elevated blood sugar levels. This disruption in blood sugar regulation can contribute to increased risk of developing type 2 diabetes and other metabolic disorders.

The Impact on Overall Well-being

Quality sleep is crucial for our overall well-being, impacting various aspects of our lives. When we consistently experience restful rejuvenation, we reap a multitude of benefits.

Cognitive Function: Adequate sleep supports optimal cognitive function, including attention, concentration, memory, and problem-solving abilities. It enhances our ability to learn and process information, allowing us to perform at our best.

Emotional Well-being: Sleep plays a vital role in regulating our emotions and mood. Sufficient sleep helps balance the production of hormones and neurotransmitters that influence our emotional state. When we are well-rested, we are better equipped to manage stress, regulate our emotions, and maintain a positive outlook.

Physical Health: Quality sleep is essential for physical health and vitality. During sleep, our bodies undergo crucial restorative processes, including tissue repair, muscle growth, and hormone regulation. It contributes to a strengthened immune system, improved cardiovascular health, and optimal metabolic function.

Strategies for Restful Rejuvenation

To optimize the connection between blood sugar stability and quality sleep, adopting strategies that promote both is essential.

Maintain a Consistent Sleep Schedule: Establish a regular sleep routine by going to bed and waking up at the same time every day, even on weekends. This helps regulate your body's internal clock and promotes better sleep quality.

Create a Restful Environment: Make your bedroom a sanctuary for sleep. Keep the room cool, dark, and quiet. Minimize distractions such as electronic devices, and consider using blackout curtains, earplugs, or white noise machines if needed.

Practice Relaxation Techniques: Incorporate relaxation techniques into your bedtime routine to promote relaxation and prepare your body for sleep. This can include deep breathing exercises, meditation, gentle stretching, or taking a warm bath.

Promote Blood Sugar Balance: Adopting a balanced diet that includes whole foods, fiber-rich carbohydrates, lean proteins, and healthy fats can help stabilize blood sugar levels. Avoiding heavy meals close to bedtime and limiting caffeine and alcohol consumption can also support better sleep quality.

Emotional Narratives of Transformed Sleep Patterns and Waking Up Refreshed

Samantha's Journey to Restful Nights

Samantha had been experiencing chronic insomnia for years, leaving her exhausted and emotionally drained. Determined to find a solution, she implemented a consistent bedtime routine. She created a calm and comfortable sleep environment by keeping her bedroom dark, cool, and free from distractions.

Samantha incorporated relaxation techniques such as meditation and deep breathing exercises before bed to calm her mind and prepare for sleep. With time and consistency, Samantha's sleep patterns improved significantly. She woke up feeling refreshed, and the newfound energy positively influenced her mood, productivity, and overall well-being.

Mike's Transformation from Night Owl to Early Riser

Mike had always considered himself a night owl, staying up late and struggling to wake up in the morning. Realizing the impact of his sleep habits on his daily life, he decided to shift his schedule and prioritize consistent sleep patterns. Mike gradually adjusted his bedtime, ensuring he got the recommended hours of sleep each night.

He also established a morning routine that included exposure to natural light, exercise, and a healthy breakfast. The transformation was remarkable, as Mike found himself waking up naturally and feeling rejuvenated. His increased energy and alertness throughout the day led to improved focus and productivity.

Emily's Recovery from Sleep Deprivation

Emily had been experiencing sleep deprivation due to a demanding work schedule and high levels of stress. Recognizing the toll it was taking on her emotional well-being, she made significant changes to restore healthy sleep patterns.

Emily practiced stress management techniques, such as journaling and engaging in relaxing activities before bed. She also established a consistent sleep schedule, prioritizing the recommended hours of sleep each night. As her sleep improved, Emily noticed a profound shift in her emotional state.

She felt more resilient, emotionally balanced, and better equipped to cope with daily challenges. Restored sleep became the foundation for her overall mental and emotional well-being.

Jacob's Journey to Conquering Nightmares

Jacob had been plagued by recurring nightmares, which resulted in disturbed sleep and fear of going to bed. Seeking relief, he sought professional help and implemented strategies to address his nightmares. Jacob practiced relaxation techniques and created a calming bedtime routine.

He also incorporated soothing activities before sleep, such as reading or listening to calming music. Gradually, Jacob's nightmares diminished, and he experienced peaceful and uninterrupted sleep. Overjoyed by this transformation, he awakened each morning with a newfound sense of calm and optimism.

Chapter 7

Culinary Delights without Restraint: Savoring the Journey

Food is not only a source of nourishment but also a means of pleasure, connection, and self-expression. By delving into the principles of mindful eating and embracing a balanced approach, we uncover heartfelt accounts of individuals who have found true harmony in their relationship with food.

The Pitfalls of Calorie Counting and Restrictive Diets

Traditional approaches to nutrition often involve strict calorie counting or restrictive diets, which can create a sense of deprivation and disconnect from the joy of eating. While these methods may produce short-term results, they can be challenging to sustain and may have negative effects on mental and emotional well-being.

Calorie counting can lead to an unhealthy fixation on numbers, promoting a mindset of restriction and guilt. It can also overlook the importance of nutrient density and overall food quality. Restrictive diets, on the other hand, often eliminate entire food groups, potentially leading to nutrient deficiencies and an unbalanced relationship with food.

Embracing Mindful Eating

Mindful eating offers an alternative approach, emphasizing the importance of being fully present and attentive to the entire eating experience. It encourages us to cultivate a deeper connection with our bodies, honor our hunger and fullness cues, and savor the flavors, textures, and aromas of our meals.

By practicing mindful eating, we can develop a greater sense of self-awareness, make conscious food choices, and foster a positive relationship with food. It allows us to listen to our body's needs, enjoy a wide variety of foods, and find satisfaction in every bite.

Heartfelt Accounts of Individuals Finding Balance and Pleasure in Their Food Choices

These personal narratives showcase individuals who have learned to trust their bodies' signals, let go of guilt and judgment, and approach food with joy and gratitude. They have discovered that nourishing themselves goes beyond the physical aspect—it encompasses emotional and social well-being as well.

Sarah's Journey to Food Freedom

Sarah had spent years counting calories and following rigid diet plans in an effort to maintain her weight. However, she realized that her relationship with food had become stressful and joyless. Determined to find a healthier approach, Sarah embraced intuitive eating.

She learned to listen to her body's hunger and fullness cues and focused on nourishing herself with wholesome, satisfying meals. By giving herself permission to enjoy a wide variety of foods in moderation, Sarah found balance and pleasure in her food choices. Her renewed sense of freedom and joy around meals contributed to improved overall well-being and a positive relationship with food.

Mark's Discovery of Mindful Eating

Mark had always rushed through meals, barely taking the time to savor the flavors and textures of the food. This changed when he discovered the concept of mindful eating. Mark began to approach his meals with intention and awareness, savoring each bite and paying attention to the sensations and tastes.

By fully engaging his senses during meals, Mark found a newfound appreciation for the culinary experience. He discovered that being present and mindful while eating not only enhanced his enjoyment of food but also helped him make healthier choices based on his body's needs.

Emily's Embrace of Balanced Indulgence

Emily had struggled with guilt and shame around indulging in her favorite foods. She often felt trapped in a cycle of strict dieting followed by binge eating. Seeking a more sustainable approach, Emily decided to embrace balanced indulgence. Instead of depriving herself of her favorite treats, she learned to savor them in moderation, fully enjoying the experience without guilt.

By incorporating a variety of nourishing foods alongside occasional indulgences, Emily found balance and pleasure in her food choices. This shift in mindset allowed her to break free from the restrictive dieting mentality and foster a healthier relationship with food.

James' Culinary Exploration and Adventure

James had always been intrigued by the diverse flavors and cuisines of the world. However, he had previously restricted himself to a narrow range of foods due to dietary rules and fears. Ready for a change, James decided to embark on a culinary exploration.

He started trying new foods, experimenting with different flavors, and embracing a more adventurous approach to eating. By expanding his palate and allowing himself to experience the joy of diverse and delicious meals, James discovered a world of culinary delight.

His newfound openness to food not only brought him pleasure but also provided a rich cultural experience.

Strategies for Savoring the Journey

To cultivate a balanced and pleasurable relationship with food, several strategies can be employed:

Practice Mindful Eating: Slow down, savor each bite, and engage all your senses while eating. Pay attention to the flavors, textures, and satisfaction that food brings.

Honor Hunger and Fullness: Listen to your body's signals of hunger and fullness. Eat when you're hungry, and stop when you're comfortably satisfied.

Emphasize Nutrient Density: Choose whole, unprocessed foods that provide a wide range of nutrients. Focus on nourishing your body with quality ingredients while still enjoying indulgences in moderation.

Cultivate Food Pleasure: Seek out foods that genuinely bring you joy and satisfaction. Allow yourself to enjoy your favorite flavors and dishes without guilt.

Foster a Positive Food Environment: Surround yourself with a supportive food environment that promotes balance and nourishment. Engage in meal planning, cooking, and sharing meals with loved ones to enhance the enjoyment of food.

Chapter 8
Embrace Lasting Change: A Lifetime of Wellness

The Power of Positive Habits

Positive habits are the foundation of long-term well-being. They are the small, consistent actions that we integrate into our daily lives to support our health and happiness. When it comes to blood sugar management, positive habits play a pivotal role in achieving and maintaining stable levels.

By incorporating habits such as mindful eating, regular physical activity, stress management techniques, and quality sleep into our routines, we create a framework for optimal blood sugar balance. These habits not only impact our immediate health but also have far-reaching effects on our long-term wellness and vitality.

Stories of Personal Growth and Transformation

Sarah's Journey to Empowered Health

Sarah had struggled with fluctuating blood sugar levels for years, which negatively impacted her energy levels, mood, and overall well-being. Determined to take control of her health, she embarked on a journey of sustained glucose management.

By adopting a balanced diet consisting of whole foods, complex carbohydrates, and regular meals, Sarah was able to stabilize her blood sugar levels. As a result, she experienced increased energy, mental clarity, and emotional stability. Sarah's newfound empowerment through glucose management fueled her personal growth, allowing her to pursue her passions and embrace a vibrant and fulfilling life.

David's Transformation from Fatigue to Vitality

David had long battled with chronic fatigue, which hindered his ability to fully engage in life's opportunities. Recognizing the impact of his blood sugar levels on his energy levels, he committed himself to sustained glucose management.

Through regular exercise, portion control, and mindful eating, David was able to stabilize his blood sugar levels and reclaim his vitality. As his energy levels soared, David found himself more motivated, productive, and open to personal growth. He embarked on new endeavors, cultivated meaningful relationships, and embraced a life of vitality that he never thought possible.

Emma's Emotional Resilience and Mental Clarity

Emma had experienced erratic blood sugar levels that often led to mood swings, brain fog, and emotional instability. Determined to find balance, she focused on sustained glucose management through a well-rounded diet and consistent meal timings.

As her blood sugar levels stabilized, Emma noticed a remarkable improvement in her emotional resilience and mental clarity. She was better equipped to handle stress, make rational decisions, and maintain a positive mindset. This newfound emotional stability propelled her personal growth journey, allowing her to pursue personal and professional goals with confidence and clarity.

Michael's Journey to Self-Discovery

Michael had struggled with weight management and low self-esteem, which hindered his personal growth and self-discovery. Recognizing the impact of glucose management on weight and emotional well-being, he adopted a holistic approach to his health.

Through balanced nutrition, regular physical activity, and mindful eating, Michael achieved sustained glucose management. As his weight stabilized and his energy levels increased, he experienced a newfound sense of self-confidence and self-discovery. Michael's personal growth journey expanded beyond his physical health, transforming his mindset and empowering him to embrace new opportunities and achieve personal fulfillment.

These individuals have recognized the importance of positive habits in their lives and have made a commitment to embrace lasting change.

Their stories highlight the challenges they faced, the lessons they learned, and the remarkable transformations they experienced. They serve as beacons of inspiration, showcasing that it is never too late to make positive changes and that through dedication and perseverance, significant improvements in health and well-being are attainable.

These individuals have witnessed not only physical transformations such as weight loss, improved energy levels, and better overall health but also profound changes in their mindset, emotional well-being, and self-confidence. Their stories remind us that the journey to wellness is a continuous one, and each step we take towards positive habits can bring us closer to our goals.

Strategies for Embracing Lasting Change

To embrace lasting change and cultivate positive habits, several strategies can be implemented:

Set Clear Goals: Define your vision for long-term well-being and set clear, achievable goals. Break them down into smaller, manageable steps to track your progress and stay motivated.

Create a Supportive Environment: Surround yourself with people who uplift and inspire you on your journey. Seek support from friends, family, or support groups who share similar goals.

Practice Consistency: Consistency is key in building positive habits. Commit to regular practice and make these habits a non-negotiable part of your daily routine.

Celebrate Small Victories: Acknowledge and celebrate your achievements along the way. Every positive step, no matter how small, contributes to your overall progress.

Stay Mindful and Adaptable: Be mindful of your habits and their effects on your well-being. Be willing to adapt and adjust your approach as needed, as we are all unique individuals with different needs and circumstances.

Conclusion
Embracing the Glucose Revolution - Your Journey Continues

As this book comes to a close, we want to empower readers to continue their journey towards health, happiness, and vitality. The knowledge and insights gained within these pages are just the beginning. It is now up to each reader to embrace the glucose revolution and apply it to their own lives.

Remember that sustainable change takes time and effort. It requires patience, commitment, and self-compassion. Embrace the small steps and celebrate every victory along the way. Stay mindful of your habits, nourish your body with balanced nutrition, move joyfully, prioritize restful sleep, and cultivate a positive relationship with food.

Seek support and surround yourself with a community of like-minded individuals who can uplift and inspire you. Share your own journey, celebrate your successes, and learn from others. Remember that everyone's path is unique, and what works for one person may not work for another. Listen to your body, trust your intuition, and make choices that align with your individual needs and goals.

The journey towards health, happiness, and vitality is a continuous one. It may have its ups and downs, but with dedication and perseverance, the rewards are immeasurable. Embrace the power of the glucose revolution and continue to prioritize your well-being.

May this book serve as a guide and a source of inspiration as you navigate the intricacies of blood sugar management. May it fuel your desire for knowledge, encourage self-reflection, and empower you to make informed choices for your health and vitality.

Your journey continues, and the possibilities are endless. Embrace the glucose revolution, and may your path be filled with abundant health, happiness, and vitality.

Grilled Lemon Herb Chicken

Ingredients:

- 4 boneless, skinless chicken breasts
- 2 lemons, juiced and zested
- 2 tablespoons olive oil
- 1 tablespoon fresh thyme, chopped
- 1 tablespoon fresh rosemary, chopped
- Salt and pepper to taste

Instructions:

- Preheat the grill to medium-high heat.
- Combine the lemon juice, lemon zest, olive oil, thyme, rosemary, salt, and pepper in a bowl.
- Place the chicken breasts in a shallow dish and pour the marinade over them, ensuring they are evenly coated.
- Grill the chicken for 6-8 minutes per side or until the internal temperature reaches 165°F (74°C).
- Remove from the grill, let it rest for a few minutes, and serve.

Roasted Salmon with Garlic and Herbs

Ingredients:

- 4 salmon fillets

- 4 cloves garlic, minced

- 2 tablespoons fresh dill, chopped

- 2 tablespoons fresh parsley, chopped

- 2 tablespoons olive oil

- Salt and pepper to taste

Instructions:

- Preheat the oven to 400°F (200°C).

- MixMix the minced garlic, dill, parsley, olive oil, salt, and pepper in a small bowl in a small bowl.

- Place the salmon fillets on a baking sheet lined with parchment paper.

- Spread the garlic and herb mixture evenly over the salmon fillets.

- Roast in the oven for about 12-15 minutes or until the salmon is cooked and flakes easily with a fork.

- Serve the roasted salmon with a side of steamed vegetables or a salad.

Quinoa and Vegetable Stir-Fry

Ingredients:

- 1 cup quinoa
- 2 cups water or vegetable broth
- 2 tablespoons sesame oil
- 2 cloves garlic, minced
- 1 red bell pepper, sliced
- 1 cup broccoli florets
- 1 cup snap peas
- 1 carrot, julienned
- 2 tablespoons soy sauce
- 1 tablespoon rice vinegar
- Salt and pepper to taste

Instructions:

- Rinse the quinoa under cold water and drain.

- In a saucepan, bring the water or vegetable broth to a boil. Add the quinoa, reduce the heat, cover, and simmer for about 15-20 minutes until the liquid is absorbed and the quinoa is tender.

- Heat the sesame oil over medium-high heat in a large skillet or wok. Add the minced garlic and cook for about 1 minute until fragrant.

- Add the sliced bell pepper, broccoli florets, snap peas, and julienned carrot to the skillet. Stir-fry for 4-5 minutes until the vegetables are crisp-tender.

- Whisk together the soy sauce, rice vinegar, salt, and pepper in a small bowl. Pour the sauce over the vegetables and stir-fry for 2-3 minutes.

- Add the cooked quinoa to the skillet and toss everything together until well combined.

- Serve the quinoa and vegetable stir-fry hot.

Mediterranean Salad with Grilled Chicken

Ingredients:

- 2 boneless, skinless chicken breasts
- 4 cups mixed salad greens
- 1 cup cherry tomatoes, halved
- 1 cucumber, diced
- 1/2 red onion, thinly sliced
- 1/4 cup Kalamata olives, pitted and halved
- 1/4 cup feta cheese, crumbled
- 2 tablespoons extra-virgin olive oil
- 2 tablespoons red wine vinegar
- 1 teaspoon dried oregano
- Salt and pepper to taste

Instructions:

- Preheat the grill to medium-high heat.
- Season the chicken breasts with salt, pepper, and dried oregano.
- Grill the chicken for 6-8 minutes per side or until the internal temperature reaches 165°F (74°C). Let it rest for a few minutes before slicing.

- Combine the salad greens, cherry tomatoes, cucumber, red onion, Kalamata olives, and feta cheese in a large bowl.

- Whisk together the extra-virgin olive oil, red wine vinegar, salt, and pepper in a small bowl to make the dressing.

- Add the grilled chicken slices to the salad and drizzle the dressing.

- Toss everything together gently until well coated. Serve the Mediterranean salad immediately.

Baked Sweet Potato with Black Beans and Avocado

Ingredients:

- 2 medium sweet potatoes
- 1 can black beans, rinsed and drained
- 1 avocado, diced
- 1/4 cup chopped fresh cilantro
- 2 tablespoons lime juice
- 1 tablespoon olive oil
- 1/2 teaspoon ground cumin
- Salt and pepper to taste

Instructions:

- Preheat the oven to 400°F (200°C).
- Pierce the sweet potatoes with a fork and place them on a baking sheet.
- Bake the sweet potatoes for about 45-50 minutes or until tender.
- Combine the black beans, diced avocado, chopped cilantro, lime juice, olive oil, cumin, salt, and pepper in a bowl.
- Once the sweet potatoes are cooked, slice them open and fluff the flesh with a fork.

- Spoon the black bean and avocado mixture over the sweet potatoes.

- Serve the baked sweet potatoes with black beans and avocado as a delicious and satisfying meal.

Egg and Vegetable Frittata

Ingredients:

- 6 large eggs
- 1/4 cup milk (can be dairy or non-dairy)
- 1 tablespoon olive oil
- 1 onion, diced
- 1 bell pepper, diced
- 1 zucchini, diced
- 1 cup spinach leaves
- Salt and pepper to taste

Instructions:

- Preheat the oven to 350°F (175°C).
- Whisk together the eggs, milk, salt, and pepper in a bowl.
- Heat the olive oil in an oven-safe skillet over medium heat.
- Add the diced onion, bell pepper, and zucchini to the skillet. Sauté for about 5 minutes until the vegetables are tender.
- Add the spinach leaves to the skillet and cook until wilted.

- Pour the egg mixture over the vegetables in the skillet and gently stir to distribute the vegetables evenly.

- Cook for 2-3 minutes until the edges of the frittata start to set.

- Transfer the skillet to the preheated oven and bake for 15-20 minutes until the frittata is set and golden.

- Remove from the oven, let it cool for a few minutes, then slice and serve.

Lentil and Vegetable Soup

Ingredients:

- 1 cup dried lentils, rinsed
- 1 onion, diced
- 2 carrots, diced
- 2 celery stalks, diced
- 3 cloves garlic, minced
- 4 cups vegetable broth
- 1 can diced tomatoes
- 1 teaspoon cumin
- 1 teaspoon paprika
- Salt and pepper to taste
- Fresh parsley, chopped (for garnish)

Instructions:

- In a large pot, heat olive oil over medium heat.
- Add the diced onion, carrots, celery, and minced garlic. Sauté for about 5 minutes until the vegetables are slightly softened.
- Add the pot's rinsed lentils, vegetable broth, diced tomatoes, cumin, paprika, salt, and pepper.

- Bring the soup to a boil, then reduce the heat to low, cover, and simmer for 25-30 minutes until the lentils are tender.

- Taste and adjust the seasonings if needed.

- Ladle the lentil and vegetable soup into bowls and garnish with fresh parsley before serving.

Berry Spinach Salad with Balsamic Vinaigrette

Ingredients:

- 4 cups baby spinach leaves
- 1 cup mixed berries (strawberries, blueberries, raspberries)
- 1/4 cup crumbled goat cheese
- 1/4 cup chopped almonds
- 2 tablespoons balsamic vinegar
- 1 tablespoon extra-virgin olive oil
- 1 teaspoon honey
- Salt and pepper to taste

Instructions:

- Combine the baby spinach leaves, mixed berries, crumbled goat cheese, and chopped almonds in a large salad bowl.
- Whisk together the balsamic vinegar, extra-virgin olive oil, honey, salt, and pepper in a small bowl to make the dressing.
- Drizzle the dressing over the salad and toss gently to coat all the ingredients.
- Serve the berry spinach salad as a refreshing and nutritious side dish or main course.

Oven-Roasted Vegetables

Ingredients:

Assorted vegetables of your choice (e.g., carrots, bell peppers, zucchini, eggplant, cherry tomatoes)

2 tablespoons olive oil

1 teaspoon dried herbs (such as thyme, rosemary, or oregano)

Salt and pepper to taste

Instructions:

- Preheat the oven to 425°F (220°C).

- Wash and chop the vegetables into bite-sized pieces.

- Toss the vegetables with olive oil, dried herbs, salt, and pepper in a large bowl until evenly coated.

- Spread the vegetables in a single layer on a baking sheet.

- Roast in the oven for about 25-30 minutes, stirring once or twice, until the vegetables are tender and caramelized.

- Remove from the oven and serve the oven-roasted vegetables as a delicious and colorful side dish.

Greek Yogurt Parfait with Berries and Nuts

Ingredients:

- 1 cup Greek yogurt
- 1 cup mixed berries (strawberries, blueberries, raspberries)
- 2 tablespoons honey
- 2 tablespoons chopped nuts (almonds, walnuts, or pistachios)

Instructions:

- Layer the Greek yogurt, mixed berries, honey, and chopped nuts in a glass or a bowl.
- Repeat the layers until all the ingredients are used, ending with a sprinkle of nuts.
- Serve the Greek yogurt parfait immediately, or refrigerate for later enjoyment.

10 Days Meal Plan

Day 1

- **Breakfast:** Vegetable omelet with 3 eggs, spinach, bell peppers, and mushrooms.

- **Snack:** Greek yogurt with mixed berries.

- **Lunch:** Quinoa and vegetable stir-fry with tofu.

- **Snack:** Carrot sticks with hummus.

- **Dinner:** Baked salmon with roasted asparagus and a side salad.

- **Dessert:** Baked apple slices sprinkled with cinnamon.

Day 2

- **Breakfast:** Overnight oats made with rolled oats, almond milk, chia seeds, and sliced almonds and berries.

- **Snack:** Celery sticks with almond butter.

- **Lunch:** Lentil and vegetable soup with a side of mixed greens.

- **Snack:** Hard-boiled eggs.

- **Dinner:** Grilled lemon herb chicken with quinoa and steamed broccoli.

- **Dessert:** Dark chocolate squares.

Day 3

- **Breakfast:** Avocado toast on whole grain bread topped with cherry tomatoes and a sprinkle of feta cheese.

- **Snack:** Apple slices with almond butter.

- **Lunch:** Mediterranean salad with grilled chicken.

- **Snack:** Mixed nuts.

- **Dinner:** Turkey meatballs with zucchini noodles and marinara sauce.

- **Dessert:** Mixed berry smoothie made with Greek yogurt and a drizzle of honey.

Day 4

- **Breakfast:** Veggie scramble made with eggs, bell peppers, onions, and spinach.

- **Snack:** Cottage cheese with sliced peaches.

- **Lunch:** Quinoa and black bean salad with diced tomatoes, cucumbers, and a squeeze of lime juice.

- **Snack:** Roasted chickpeas.

- **Dinner:** Baked sweet potato with black beans, avocado, and steamed broccoli.

- **Dessert:** Chia seed pudding with coconut milk and fresh berries.

Day 5

- **Breakfast:** Greek yogurt parfait with layers of yogurt, granola, and mixed berries.

- **Snack:** Sliced cucumbers with tzatziki dip.

- **Lunch:** Grilled chicken Caesar salad with romaine lettuce, cherry tomatoes, and Parmesan cheese.

- **Snack:** Rice cakes with almond butter.

- **Dinner:** Stir-fried tofu with mixed vegetables served over brown rice.

- **Dessert:** Baked pear with a sprinkle of cinnamon.

Day 6

- **Breakfast:** Spinach and mushroom frittata with a side of sliced avocado.

- **Snack:** Baby carrots with hummus.

- **Lunch:** Quinoa-stuffed bell peppers topped with melted mozzarella cheese.

- **Snack:** Greek yogurt with crushed almonds.

- **Dinner:** Baked cod with roasted Brussels sprouts and a quinoa salad.

- **Dessert:** Mixed fruit salad.

Day 7

- **Breakfast:** Berry smoothie bowl topped with granola and coconut flakes.

- **Snack:** Hard-boiled eggs.

- **Lunch:** Lentil and vegetable curry served over brown rice.

- **Snack:** Celery sticks with almond butter.

- **Dinner:** Grilled shrimp skewers with grilled vegetables and a side of quinoa.

- **Dessert:** Dark chocolate-covered strawberries.

Day 8

- **Breakfast:** Oatmeal with sliced bananas, almond butter, and a sprinkle of cinnamon.

- **Snack:** Mixed nuts.

- **Lunch:** Greek salad with grilled chicken.

- **Snack:** Rice cakes with avocado spread.

- **Dinner:** Baked turkey breast with roasted sweet potatoes and steamed green beans.

- **Dessert:** Yogurt parfait with layers of yogurt, granola, and sliced peaches.

Day 9

- **Breakfast:** Vegetable and goat cheese omelet.

- **Snack:** Sliced apples with peanut butter.

- **Lunch:** Chickpea and vegetable wrap with whole grain tortilla.

- **Snack:** Cottage cheese with mixed berries.

- **Dinner:** Baked salmon with quinoa pilaf and roasted asparagus.

- **Dessert:** Baked apple slices with a sprinkle of cinnamon.

Day 10

- **Breakfast:** Spinach and feta cheese scramble.

- **Snack:** Carrot sticks with hummus.

- **Lunch:** Quinoa and black bean bowl with avocado, tomatoes, and a squeeze of lime.

- **Snack:** Greek yogurt with honey and crushed almonds.

- **Dinner:** Grilled chicken with roasted vegetables and a side salad.

- **Dessert:** Mixed berry smoothie with a dollop of Greek yogurt.

Monday	Breakfast	Lunch	Dinner

Tuesday	Breakfast	Lunch	Dinner

Wednesday	Breakfast	Lunch	Dinner

Thursday	Breakfast	Lunch	Dinner

Friday	Breakfast	Lunch	Dinner

Saturday	Breakfast	Lunch	Dinner

Sunday	Breakfast	Lunch	Dinner

Monday	Breakfast	Lunch	Dinner

Tuesday	Breakfast	Lunch	Dinner

Wednesday	Breakfast	Lunch	Dinner

Thursday	Breakfast	Lunch	Dinner

Friday	Breakfast	Lunch	Dinner

Saturday	Breakfast	Lunch	Dinner

Sunday	Breakfast	Lunch	Dinner

<table>
<tr><td rowspan="2">Monday</td><td>Breakfast</td><td>Lunch</td><td>Dinner</td></tr>
<tr><td></td><td></td><td></td></tr>
</table>

<table>
<tr><td rowspan="2">Tuesday</td><td>Breakfast</td><td>Lunch</td><td>Dinner</td></tr>
<tr><td></td><td></td><td></td></tr>
</table>

<table>
<tr><td rowspan="2">Wednesday</td><td>Breakfast</td><td>Lunch</td><td>Dinner</td></tr>
<tr><td></td><td></td><td></td></tr>
</table>

<table>
<tr><td rowspan="2">Thursday</td><td>Breakfast</td><td>Lunch</td><td>Dinner</td></tr>
<tr><td></td><td></td><td></td></tr>
</table>

<table>
<tr><td rowspan="2">Friday</td><td>Breakfast</td><td>Lunch</td><td>Dinner</td></tr>
<tr><td></td><td></td><td></td></tr>
</table>

<table>
<tr><td rowspan="2">Saturday</td><td>Breakfast</td><td>Lunch</td><td>Dinner</td></tr>
<tr><td></td><td></td><td></td></tr>
</table>

<table>
<tr><td rowspan="2">Sunday</td><td>Breakfast</td><td>Lunch</td><td>Dinner</td></tr>
<tr><td></td><td></td><td></td></tr>
</table>

Monday	Breakfast	Lunch	Dinner

Tuesday	Breakfast	Lunch	Dinner

Wednesday	Breakfast	Lunch	Dinner

Thursday	Breakfast	Lunch	Dinner

Friday	Breakfast	Lunch	Dinner

Saturday	Breakfast	Lunch	Dinner

Sunday	Breakfast	Lunch	Dinner

Monday	Breakfast	Lunch	Dinner

Tuesday	Breakfast	Lunch	Dinner

Wednesday	Breakfast	Lunch	Dinner

Thursday	Breakfast	Lunch	Dinner

Friday	Breakfast	Lunch	Dinner

Saturday	Breakfast	Lunch	Dinner

Sunday	Breakfast	Lunch	Dinner

Monday	Breakfast	Lunch	Dinner

Tuesday	Breakfast	Lunch	Dinner

Wednesday	Breakfast	Lunch	Dinner

Thursday	Breakfast	Lunch	Dinner

Friday	Breakfast	Lunch	Dinner

Saturday	Breakfast	Lunch	Dinner

Sunday	Breakfast	Lunch	Dinner

Monday	Breakfast	Lunch	Dinner

Tuesday	Breakfast	Lunch	Dinner

Wednesday	Breakfast	Lunch	Dinner

Thursday	Breakfast	Lunch	Dinner

Friday	Breakfast	Lunch	Dinner

Saturday	Breakfast	Lunch	Dinner

Sunday	Breakfast	Lunch	Dinner

Monday	Breakfast	Lunch	Dinner

Tuesday	Breakfast	Lunch	Dinner

Wednesday	Breakfast	Lunch	Dinner

Thursday	Breakfast	Lunch	Dinner

Friday	Breakfast	Lunch	Dinner

Saturday	Breakfast	Lunch	Dinner

Sunday	Breakfast	Lunch	Dinner

Monday	Breakfast	Lunch	Dinner

Tuesday	Breakfast	Lunch	Dinner

Wednesday	Breakfast	Lunch	Dinner

Thursday	Breakfast	Lunch	Dinner

Friday	Breakfast	Lunch	Dinner

Saturday	Breakfast	Lunch	Dinner

Sunday	Breakfast	Lunch	Dinner

Monday	Breakfast	Lunch	Dinner

Tuesday	Breakfast	Lunch	Dinner

Wednesday	Breakfast	Lunch	Dinner

Thursday	Breakfast	Lunch	Dinner

Friday	Breakfast	Lunch	Dinner

Saturday	Breakfast	Lunch	Dinner

Sunday	Breakfast	Lunch	Dinner

www.ingramcontent.com/pod-product-compliance
Lightning Source LLC
Chambersburg PA
CBHW051829250726
48659CB00005B/1743